<u>Optimize</u>

Steps to Lose Weight, Fight Disease and Maximize Mental and Physical Performance

Matthew Kansy, RD

Optimize

Independently Published

Copyright © 2019, Matthew Kansy, RD

Published in the United States of America

180221-599591-4
ISBN: 9781091251731

Here's What's Inside...

Introduction

Optimize!

As a dietitian for the past twenty years, I've come to realize that a nutritional approach alone wasn't always addressing my clients' needs to achieve the health and vitality. This forced me to take the time to step back and develop a better understanding of the underpinnings of most modern-day health issues.

I realized that I needed to educate myself in other areas in order to develop a better picture of how lifestyle choices influence health, well-being, and performance. By addressing the major components of lifestyle (nutrition, sleep, physical activity, mindset, and stress-reducing strategies) I started to experience significantly better results with my clients. I was then able to help individuals progress with their health and wellness and performance goals much faster with longer-lasting results than when I strictly focused on nutrition.

Modern-day life can be an amazing experience for us all. With advancements in technology and science, we are capable of living and experiencing so many amazing things! We are no longer required to do all of the daily labors of our ancestors and modern-day conveniences have allowed us to allocate our time for other more desirable activities. These advancements have made life much better in some sense, but the truth is they have also created some significant problems for us as well.

Take something as simple as the electric light bulb. When Thomas Edison created this amazing invention, he probably had no idea how he was going to change humanity forever. With his invention, we began to stay up past sunset and get up before sunrise, throwing us off our natural circadian rhythm. That was a catalyst, among others, that began to alter our natural behaviors and ultimately disrupt our natural state of being.

As human beings, we've spent over two-hundred-thousand years evolving and living around the rhythm of the rising and setting sun. And in such a short amount of time, just over 100 years, we have advanced our technology so rapidly that our bodies and minds have not been able to adapt quickly enough to remain as healthy as we are capable of doing. We have turned away from a diet consisting entirely of real nutrient dense foods and have embraced highly palatable, cheap, nutrient poor, processed, industrialized, engineered foods. Additionally, the amount of daily physical activity that we used to get each day has also been compromised as a result of advancements in transportation and other time-saving conveniences. No longer do we have to physically engage ourselves on a daily basis in order to accomplish the chores of everyday life.

And, it doesn't stop there. We are now being bombarded continually with stressful stimulation and complex scenarios every second of every day--relationships, money, advertisements, food, social media, computers, technology, noise, light, chemicals and social isolation -- just to name a few. Everything is so vibrant and intense, and all those stimuli affect our psyche. We're not able to tune out from these things. Our lack of mindfulness and increasing stress, anxiety, and depression are a result not only of biological imbalances (caused by a poor diet, lack of physical activity and poor sleep), but from overstimulation that we can't keep up with, never mind turn off.

But, there is a solution. By putting things into place (proper nutrition, good sleep strategies, the right amount of physical activity, and stress-management strategies), we are able to find and create balance and counteract these pitfalls of modern-day life.

Although moving up to the mountains, living off the land, and removing ourselves from modern-day stressors and technology would probably help a lot of people find health and wellbeing; I am proposing much simpler countermeasures to help offset the negative impacts of today's environment. It's about taking the best of technology and its advancements and using them as tools without becoming enslaved to them. It's about using the wisdom and practices of our ancestors in conjunction with these advancements in order to find harmony and balance, ultimately leading to optimal health and happiness.

I've wanted to get the information and resources in this book out there so that it can help more people. I've found the strategies, and my approach has been eye-opening and effective, not only for myself and my family, but also for my clients.

To optimize ourselves and be the best we can be mentally and physically, we must work on our foundation. We must work on the fundamentals of how the human body and brain evolved over hundreds of thousands of years -- without neglecting the best of what modern-day technology and advancements have brought us. We need to establish basic countermeasures and balance in our lives associated with nutrition, physical movement, sleep, and stress-management strategies.

I hope that this book convinces you that you're not broken and that the most basic of lifestyle practices can lead to significant change as it relates to your health and happiness. All of the latest gadgets and supplements that are out there, all the commercials trying to convince you that you are broken and that you need their product to be better are sales gimmicks to trick you into purchasing their products or services. The truth is that it's our choice to put our own health and well-being first.

In this book, I have outlined the fundamental steps needed to optimize your performance. Consider this, greater than ninety percent of all the reasons we go to do the doctor, and greater than ninety percent of all pharmaceuticals that are on the market, are to address our lifestyle habits. Understand that by addressing those lifestyle habits, we can greatly reduce and potentially eliminate our need for medications and unplanned visits to the doctor.

To your optimal health!

Matt

P.S. In the back of this book, there are a few pages for you to take notes. Please take advantage of this as you read. Jot down the thoughts, ideas and goals that will help create success.

The Pitfalls of Modern Life

I remember back in the '70s when my mother came home with my very first frozen dinner. She bought it because it was the hot new trend meant to provide a meal without the time and hassle typically required. This was a convenience that freed her to do other things, but the unfortunate result was this simple meal prep neglected our mutual need for nutrition. From birth to death, as we move through life, we are faced with challenges. In most cases how we deal with these situations is already laid out for us -- either by our parents, teachers, other family members, friends, or society as a whole. As our society is influenced by our technological advancements, we get swept up in the idea that we have created something better than what nature has provided.

When we are faced with social challenges that need to be addressed, we have choices. Unfortunately, we tend to choose the easiest or more socially accepted option rather than traditional or more options that are more.

Most people take whatever is the easiest approach, or whatever everybody else is doing. Say, for instance, "I don't have enough time to cook, so what am I going to do? Go through a drive-through, graze out of a bag or throw a frozen meal into the oven." Sure, that addresses the immediate need, "I don't have time to cook, and I need to eat." We end up feeding ourselves, but we neglect the nourishment that is so desperately needed for optimal health. Grabbing things on the go becomes a habit, and before you know it, you are eating out of a bag more than you care to admit.

Another problem is that all these processed foods are so hyper-palatable. They are foods that are designed to stimulate your taste buds and brain. These things are created to stimulate the pleasure centers of the brain. Either with sugar, salt or some other hyper-palatable substance that forces you to go, "Wow. That's amazing." It lights up your taste buds and your dopamine receptors. These products not only over stimulate the taste buds, rendering natural real foods dissatisfying, but are also scientifically proven to be addictive. If you have ever attempted to reduce your intake of sugar and/or refined grains, you might know what I am talking about. It's very easy to fall into these traps because of the simple fact that we are like alcoholics in the bar of life! We are inundated with these products and we have established lifestyle habits and prioritize other things over the optimal choices for our bodies and brains.

If you look at the pitfalls of modern-day society, the choices that we make over time lead to an imbalance of how humans have evolved to live and survive-- to live like a human being from a natural perspective, rather than a manufactured, industrialized, convenience perspective.

Back in the seventies, when I received that first frozen meal, I was like, "Wow, that's super tasty." But then, as you get used to the higher levels of salt and artificial flavor enhancers, the palate and taste buds adjust to prefer those flavors over more natural ones. I can recall the amount of time my mother and grandparents spent in the kitchen cooking, and the times you heard of someone spending all day in the kitchen making tomato sauce. Compare that to how little time we spend in the kitchen preparing food these days

Back in the 1950s, the national average of time spent in the kitchen for dinner alone was two-and-a-half hours-- every day in the kitchen, to prepare one meal! Right now, if you spend two-and-a-half hours in your kitchen over the span of a whole week that can be considered a lot.

Granted, there are people out there who are still spending a lot of time in the kitchen, and with the new surge of culinary shows and fancy gadgets it can become a competitive event. We feel that we have to do something special. The truth is, this increase in culinary television shows has actually reduced our time in the kitchen and increased the amount of time we spend in front of the TV. Making a simple meal consisting of vegetables, a starch and some form of protein is not enough. We have to be competitive and say that we did something super-fancy or used some unique ingredient so we can post it on Instagram and get likes.

It is not uncommon for people to stop cooking because they are intimidated or become frustrated with the equipment they have or can no longer tolerate dull knives. It's all a matter of perspective and priorities. Consider the challenge of taking someone who has lived a life of convenience, but doing things that they were indoctrinated to do from a young age. Turning them around and teaching them how to cook, move their body, or place emphasis on quality sleep can be a very difficult in most cases. It is so foreign to them yet, from an ancestral perspective, it's the most natural state to live in.

Another downside to our modern lifestyle is our emphasis on calories. There is so much sugar-laden food everywhere we turn. We've been told the more we eat, the more we weigh.

The less we eat, the less we weigh. It's all about calories in, calories out. But, in truth, it's not. Calories certainly play a role, but first and foremost, food quality is extremely important.

We have one-hundred-calorie snack packs of cookies, chips, baked goods, and so on. We have developed the mind-set that as long as long as we don't go over our calories, we are doing okay. This is completely ignoring the nutritional aspect of food and the hormonal and inflammatory chaos that poor quality food can create. Do you think two hundred calories of sugar is the same as two hundred calories of chicken or butter? How your body responds to each of these foods, hormonally, digestively, and chemically, is vastly different.

The signaling to the brain and body from the consumption of carbohydrates, proteins and fats are radically different from each other. It's remarkable how easily we are swayed to react to a sensationalized headline or news snippet that comes from an outlet that is focusing on market share rather than actual honest clear insights and accurate depiction of the science. As a society, we often look for the easiest solution for our problems and are desperate to find the quick fix to what ails us. But, as you might expect at this point in the book, real health is something that doesn't come from a pill or some fancy product, it comes from fundamental lifestyle practices that have been established by our ancestors for thousands of years.

Better Health, Better Life

To better understand how to optimize our health and performance, we need to better understand the things that are holding us back. For instance, many diseases have an inflammatory component to them. The majority of the diseases that plague our society are classified as auto-immune disorders. When we look at the terminology or the definition of auto-immune, it is actually our own immune system that is attacking the tissues of our body.

If that had always been a natural state of human evolution, then I don't think we would have survived as a species; there are relatively newer problems. By optimizing our food, physical activity, sleep, and mindset, we allow ourselves ability to lower inflammation, balance hormones, and strengthen the immune system.

When we consider the micronutrient components of nutrient dense real foods, we can't ignore the role they play in our health.

Macronutrients are the carbohydrates, proteins, and fats in our diet; micronutrients are the vitamins and minerals. When we're eating a more vegetable-based diet, with a lot of nutrient density, then we are nourishing ourselves. The difference between feeding ourselves and nourishing ourselves is the quality and nutrient density of the food we eat.

When people start adopting more lifestyle habits that are natural to the human condition, body and brain, we start to see that it will function much better. However, when we fall into the trap of modern-day conveniences and industrialized food, that's when our cells are compromised, and they can no longer continue to function the way they should.

Ten years into being a dietitian, I was adhering to the standard protocols recommended by the American Heart Association and Diabetic Association. They certainly have a lot invested in research and science, but are also strongly influenced by big pharma, the food and agriculture industry, and government. However, following those rules alone and thinking that a one-size-fits-all approach is the best way to treat people only resulted in minimal success. Saying certain nutritional choices are ideal for everybody is a big mistake, because there is such great genetic diversity. Consider how different the nutritional needs are for those who live closer versus farther from the equator.

There's no one ideal diet that works for everyone, but there are some very sound fundamentals. The only thing that I am sure of is that ALL healthy lifestyles emphasize the need for a variety of lots of vegetables in the diet. All diets should be vegetable based; not necessarily vegetarian per say, but vegetable rich with a focus on plants as a foundation. Quality animal products can also be a part of a healthy diet for many people.

Once I realized that eating per certain guidelines was compromising my health, as well as my clients' health and performance, my focus on more natural elements changed and yielded remarkable results. I now understand how much better we can perform if we nourish ourselves and use food in the correct way; optimal food as a tool --yes, a tool. I use this term because we must acknowledge what food is first and foremost. Food is essential to fuel and nourish the body, but unfortunately food is now mostly associated with pleasure. Not to say that food cannot be pleasurable, it's just that most foods are overly processed and designed for pleasure, not nutrition. Regardless of what the packaging and label might say. We use food more as a means of self-medication to deal with stress, cravings, and blood sugar swings. Yes, we need to eat and avoid hunger and function properly, but to perform mentally and physically at the highest level consider how you feed yourself pre- or a post-exercise, earlier or later in the day.

The typical American breakfast for most people is more akin to dessert rather than a nourishing meal. No wonder we fall victim to emotional eating and blood sugar swings. If we focus on nourishment rather than carbohydrates and empty calories, we significantly impact how we look, feel, and perform throughout the day.

In my early days as a dietitian, I eventually began to realize that my diet was preventing me from getting the results I wanted in my physical endeavors (cycling, running, lifting, and even yard work). I realized that I was dealing with significant blood sugar swings and was constantly grazing to help regulate it. There's a new term that we use in an almost joking manner: "Hangry." Angry and hungry smashed into one word, and now it's used in TV commercials, like it's funny or something to joke about. I suppose the reason that some of us might find it humorous is because most of us can relate. But truthfully speaking, I don't that there is anyone who really enjoys the feeling of low blood sugar. This condition is actually a sign of a malfunctioning metabolism and hormonal dis-regulation. Once I realized how my hormonal dis-regulation and blood sugar swings were affecting my state of mind, I decided to do something about it. Being a father of three young children, dealing with work related anxiety and stress, I realized that my food intake had a profound impact on how well I managed these things.

When I decided to adopt a diet of healthier, more natural nutritious foods eliminating refined grains and sugars and integrating more whole foods and natural fats, my mental state improved significantly. I slimmed down quite a bit as well and without even trying. I've never been heavy mind you, but I certainly was able to lose those ten to fifteen pounds easily enough just by focusing on the quality of my food.

I also had the auto-immune disorder eczema and debilitating seasonal allergies. I realized after just a few months that both had improved significantly by about eighty percent. It took about another year or two for the eczema to go away entirely and my allergy symptoms aren't much more than an occasional sneeze and runny nose. Keep in mind, before changing my diet, I was on steroidal creams for over a decade to treat my skin condition and taking a daily dose of allergy medication four months out of the year. When I realized the quality of my food intake had such a huge impact on my skin, that was a big turning point that led me to dig deeper into what other possible effects that my diet was having on me and my clients.

Hippocrates said it best, "all disease begins in the gut." He also made the statement, "Let food be thy medicine, and medicine be thy food." Although over two-thousand years old, these statements are about as true as can be when it comes to health and wellness associated with nutrition as we could ever have.

I would like to share five different cases with you where I helped clients modify their lifestyle habits that yielded some very satisfying results. Keep in mind that everyone is different and real change takes time, but the foundation of most illnesses and disease are rooted in one's lifestyle choices. Amazing results can be had through the proper changes in nutrition, physical movement, sleep, and stress management strategies.

Example #1

This example is a female client in her late 60s whose primary concern was her weight. She was always battling significant weight fluctuations shifting up and down fifty pounds or so for the majority of her life. By changing her mind-set around food and engaging with some simple protocols, she finally found a system that allowed her to lose the weight once and for all. As it is for most of us, her weight deeply affected her state of happiness. She realized that the dietary approaches that she was trying were not only unfulfilling, but they also weren't sustainable because of how extreme they were, for instance mostly calorie restriction and not nutritionally adequate.

Once I started working with her, I came to realize how much of a "sugarholic" she was, like so many of us are. She craved refined carbohydrates, chocolate, and sugars. She actually depended on them, to a certain extent, for her mental state. We're talking about self-medicating with food rather than using food for nourishment and sustenance.

Over time, as change began to occur, it was evident that this journey was more of a psychological shift over anything else. By helping her improve her relationship with food and her understanding how the food was being the puppet-master over her life, she started to realize the impact it was having on her physically and psychologically. From there, she was able to start to approach things in a more mindful matter.

I don't feel a dietary change should be done radically. In fact, most diets fail because one tends to take on too much too quickly creating a very disruptive and stressful state. I like to encourage small, sustainable changes. One simple step was to change the quality of chocolate that she was eating. Rather than your typical low-quality everyday chocolate, I had her switch to a higher-quality dark chocolate with a cocoa content over seventy percent, which was something that met her needs, but also something that she could savor and deeply enjoy.

Rather than eating a whole bar of chocolate, she was able to enjoy higher-quality chocolate and eat far less of it. Higher quality of chocolate with a higher cocoa content has far less sugar. (One trick is to not let the chocolate touch your teeth. Let it melt and coat your mouth.)

From there, she started looking at other sources of sugar. She was able to slowly turn down the volume knob on those cravings, by not eliminating them, but slowly finding healthier alternatives. For her, this took quite some time because I wanted her to be compassionate with herself. I didn't want her to feel deprived, as I wanted the changes to stick. Over the course of a year or so, she found herself in a completely different place. She had lost the weight she wanted to lose, and not only that, she was living a life that was sustainable and didn't feel like she was white-knuckling it and could fall off the wagon at any time.

She was more than happy with the food choices, and although she still loved her chocolate and certain other vices, they were no longer controlling her life. She's not eating them on a daily basis like she was before and now has them as occasional treats, but it took her a while to get there. It's been six or seven years now, and she's doing fantastic!

Example #2

My next client is a young mother with two small children, who was doing all of the typical things that busy mothers do these days–finding the path of least resistance when it came to feeding herself and her family. At some point she realized that short-cuts were not yielding very good results. Sure, they might seem to save time, but when once you realize the negative impact that they have on how you feel or the potential behaviors that they can cause, that saved time gets lost when it comes to their health. Eventually, through small, yet impactful changes she began to see the benefits of taking the time to do things right. In this case, the changes were making the majority of the meals utilizing real ingredients and preparing them properly.

If you are reading this and thinking to yourself, "Well, I don't have time or energy to make these radical changes," reflect back on the first client that I described to you. She made one small change one at a time--not rushing for results or taking on too much, which can cause a significant amount of stress; for her, it started with making better food choices.

As an example, let's consider the first meal of the day: breakfast. Understanding that, most American breakfasts are akin to dessert. We typically consume refined grains. These include hot or cold cereal, bagels, waffles, pancakes, Danishes, and muffins, usually with juice or toast. Many people put more sugar in their coffee than there is in ice cream. Think about that for a moment. We have this big refined sugar bomb for breakfast, and it sets us up for failure for the rest of the day. But, by just addressing one meal each day and not focusing on all of them, this client was able to make smaller changes one at a time. Once one area is mastered, then you take on the next challenge.

What this young mother found was that over time, by starting the day with more nutrient-rich foods, healthy fats and protein, she had more sustainable energy. This allowed her to eat less as she wasn't starving or reacting to a drop in her blood sugar. She was instead, consuming two to three solid nutrient-rich meals, rather than constantly grazing throughout the day.

This protocol allowed her more time to cook and take care of her kids and run errands. She found, over time, that her new dietary habits and stress-reducing techniques helped her manage the stressful work of maintaining her home and raising her children. These strategies eventually led to having more energy and more patience.

Example #3

My next client is a male corporate professional that spends a significant amount of time in his car or on a plane while living out of a suitcase four to five nights per week. His work environment is certainly stressful with that much travel. Like most "road warriors," he opted for convenience items that simply fed him rather than choosing more nourishing foods that his body and brain so desperately needed.

He also realized that all of the sitting he was doing was having an impact on his physical health. Coupled with poor dietary habits this lifestyle started to take its toll. His food choices mostly consisted of refined grains and sugars, which was having an impact on his mental state, focus, and energy levels.

We started by simply adjusting his sugar intake. There were a lot of liquid calories, such as sodas, juice, and the sugar in his coffee. Albeit not easy as first, eliminating the calories that he was drinking had a massive impact. Neither one of us actually realized how many calories these sugary drinks were adding up to each day. Never mind the impact it had on other biological systems in his body. Once conquered, we then slowly moved onto some of his food choices.

In a relatively short period of time, he started to have much better energy levels and certainly slimming in his waistline. We also incorporated some very simple bodyweight exercises and activities that he could easily do in a hotel gym or even in his room. These exercises were not only to help with weight loss, but to also counteract the negative impact of all of the sitting he was doing. He soon discovered that his daily routine also had a positive impact on his state of mind and was improving his sleep quality as well.

Putting together a very simple physical movement routine helped how he felt physically as well as improving his posture. I feel more importantly; regular physical activity is an essential component of one's psychological health. Most people think exercise is something we do to burn calories, but in truth, that's more of a secondary or tertiary effect of exercise.

An effective exercise routine is essential for keeping our body mobile and physically capable, but more importantly it is the impact that it has on our nervous system that is often overlooked. I've done a lot of work with individuals in the past with autism spectrum disorder, and when vigorous physical activity was incorporated into their daily routine, the impact that it had on their mental and physical state was nothing short of remarkable. Regular physical activity improves our ability to concentrate, learn, improves our sleep quality, digestion, as well as our sense of happiness and wellbeing. By using exercise, as for this gentleman, we found that he was able to have a better state of mind, less stress and anxiety, able to think more clearly, and get a better night's sleep.

Example#4

My next client is another example of a business professional, but in this case most of his time is spent sitting at his office desk. He has a busy home life, as well, with two young boys that are very active throughout the year with sports activities. He is in his mid-fifties now, but throughout high school and college, he was very athletic; wrestling, playing lacrosse, as well as football. For most of us, once we get out of school, sports and athletics tend to go to the wayside because of work, financial obligations and the time constraints of starting a family. Life starts to take a different trajectory and different priorities begin to surface. But even at fifty, although you're not in your twenties anymore, you can still get out there and move your body. In fact, fifty is still a very young age where just about anyone can learn to get out there and be a very active individual.

I think that's the case for many of my clients. Despite good intentions, life gets away from them. In this case, as it is common for many people, he found himself, thirty-five years later, fifty pounds overweight, having knee and back issues, and suffering from a significant lack of mobility. And, as you might be able to imagine, the cause of his decreased mobility was pain.

We started to use his diet to help not only fuel and nourish his body and brain, but to also dramatically lower the amount of unnecessary inflammation that was plaguing his system. He responded quite quickly to the dietary changes and experienced not only improved mobility, but also a drop in the amount of body fat that he was holding on to. By reducing the inflammation, it allowed him to move a little bit more freely day by day. A poor quality diet is a leading cause of systemic inflammation, which can have a detrimental effect of just about every system in the body-- not only physical discomfort, but also things like cardiovascular disease, which, by the way, is not a disease of high cholesterol, but a disease of inflammation.

When we nourish the body and reduce inflammation, we also decrease some of the risk factors associated with some of the deadliest diseases. In this individual's case, it allowed him to be more physically active, which opened the door to then embracing some of the physical activities he used to love when he was younger and be more active with his boys.

As you can imagine, there was a lot of time between his twenties and fifties that he didn't do very much of anything physical, putting his career before his personal health. His journey back was a slow progression, but eventually he got to the point where he ended up running a 5K. And things didn't stop there, he is now mountain biking and going on ski trips with his friends. He even started to help coach some of the sporting activities that his boys are playing. But, that was just the beginning of the discoveries that he was about to experience.

Of the four different areas we are going to talk about in this book, he said the one that had the most impact was his development of a daily mindfulness practice. This included breathing exercises, mindfulness, and a meditation practice to help him maintain more calmness and be more responsive to stressful situations, rather than reactive. Developing the ability to be more in tune and pay more attention to the people in his life had the biggest impact. He is now able to limit the negative impact that his inner dialogue of negativity and worry had on him.

Ninety percent of all the negativity we face actually comes from our own thoughts. Once he realized this, he was then able to better understand that his own thoughts were, in some cases, deceiving him and leading him down a thought path that was increasing his stress. He found that a simple mindfulness practice had the greatest impact on his overall health.

Example #5

Lastly, is a client that I have been working with for about a year now: She is in her early sixties, was never physically active, and had mounting health issues like suffering from ailments such as acid reflux, arthritis, and mild cardiovascular issues. By addressing certain aspects of her health and peeling the layers back slowly, we were able to make huge strides in her life, health, and sense of wellbeing.

First off, she was most definitely a sugarholic. She works in a large office building, sits for most the day, and as you can imagine, is constantly tempted by the bagels, donuts, and candy bowls that frequent such environments. These types of work atmospheres make it very, very difficult to make smart food choices. And the competitive, must-look-busy mindset keeps her from getting up from her desk to move and stretch. We first started to work on her mental strategies to enable her to combat the food temptations. It took a little while, but eventually she found it easier and easier to ignore and walk away from the candy and baked goods. In fact, she actually started up a conversation about the unnecessary food, which made an impact on the frequency and amounts that were typically available.

By simply asking the person next to her to her to keep the candy bowl on the other side of the desk, it eventually ended up in a drawer because it was too tempting for both of them. It's funny how people think they're trying to be nice by giving candy, but in the end, it's actually causing some harm.

What was most concerning with her was her lack of physical mobility. We started with very simple exercise and fundamental movement strategies. She still does them to this day, but at a more advanced level, and is doing remarkably well. The first thing I taught her to do before we started exercise was how to breathe properly. She was what we could consider a "mouth breather" and suffered from sleep apnea. So we started with some breathing exercises that utilized the nose and activates the diaphragm more. Since she works on the sixth floor of an eight-story building, the exercise program included walking up and down the stairs while trying to breathe only through her nose.

At first, she would make it up about one flight before she needed to breathe through her mouth in order to catch her breath. But, only after a few months, she eventually was able to go up and down all eight flights, while only breathing in and out through her nose. This alone has been a huge accomplishment for her and has yielded significant results. Such as improved sleep, better cardiovascular health, less stress, weight loss, and more self-confidence!

What's great about weight loss through this process is that it's much more sustainable than your typical dietary protocol. Learning new habits and addressing one thing at a time is a process of learning and understanding that once accomplished cannot be undone. Granted, one can choose to make poor choices, but if you take your time and "re-program" yourself it becomes much easier to make healthier choices for the rest of your life.

For this client, it didn't happen quickly. It occurred slowly over time, but as long as she maintains the lifestyle habits that she's adopted over the course of the past year, the weight will continue to drop, and stay off. Needless to say, I am extremely proud of her accomplishments and ambition.

Another thing that's important to realize is that her shoulder and knee issues greatly limited her physically. By improving her nutrition, we greatly reduced the harmful and unnecessary systemic inflammation from which she was suffering. By lowering the inflammation this allowed her to have a more freedom of movement because of less pain in those joints.

One of the exercises she does on a daily basis, which I think everybody should learn how to do with ease and efficiency, is some form of getting up and down from the floor. One's ability to get up from the floor is a unit of measurement that doctors use to asses an elderly patient's risk for premature death. That being said, how easy is it for you to get up and down from the floor? If you find this to be difficult, your health and longevity is at a greater risk.

Getting back to this example, one of her daily exercises was to practice getting up and down from the floor. At first, she was using props, such as a chair, sofa, or table. Now, after some practice, she can do it without any props. It took her about six months to get to the point where she didn't need assistance from anything else around her. She can do it from both sides, meaning that she can push herself up from her right side or left side. She has gained the strength and mobility in both her legs and arms to do so with much more ease.

Simply getting up and down from the floor is an amazing practice for developing strength and fitness. Some of the best exercises out there utilize this concept. Two examples are the burpee and Turkish get-up.

For her, we slowed it way down. There was fear in her of, "Oh, I don't want to get down on the floor to do that exercise." I asked, "Why not?" She replied, "Well, I might not be able to get back up." That was a shock to me to hear her say that and I knew that it needed to be addressed.

Over the course of the past year, I've done much more questioning of older clients in their 60's and 70's. Such as, "How do you feel about hopping or lightly jumping up and down a few times; or, going up and down steps without the use of the hand rail?" The look of fear they express is very enlightening. Even jumping rope, "Oh, I could never do that." They're afraid they're going to twist an ankle or not be able to get up. These are all instances of our body declining because of lack of use. Now, I'm not saying that they need to get out there and do it immediately. Obviously, they need to ease into some of these movements, given the fact that the inability to get up and down from a chair or the inability to use the stairs with confidence has a huge impact on one's quality of life.

If we maintain our ability to use the stairs, do a little hop and get up and down from the ground with ease and confidence, then we'll be much more capable as we age. But, when we are more sedentary and don't do much of anything physical on a daily basis, we lose our ability to properly function and move.

Getting back to this particular client, I was so amazed at her determination. At first, she was saying, "I don't know if I can do this!" She was genuinely scared. Having one success let to a second one. She's had so many at this point that she doesn't think anything is impossible. It takes time. She's patient with herself now. And, that is what you need to do as well, be patient and confident that change will occur.

Developing patience is absolutely essential for success. When it comes to diet and exercise, we look for the magic bullets and that success should happen immediately. This is a huge mistake. Real change takes time. When you hear ads that make statements such as, "Lose thirty pounds in thirty days", or "get six-pack abs in six weeks!" turn and run the other way. With those types of approaches, success is very rare and more than likely over time the weight will just come back on.

When we do it slow and steady, this is real change. That takes time. Now, I know that there are people out there who have amazing success stories with quick results, but for most of us this is just not reality. There are so many things in life that we've acknowledged and accepted as truths, such as that people don't become millionaires overnight; if we need to amass wealth, it takes time -- a lot of my clients in the financial industry will acknowledge that. When it comes to health and losing weight, they wanted it to happen yesterday. And I'm like, "It doesn't work that way." You have to take your time, and you have to be compassionate with yourself. You have to be patient.

Lastly, I dislike the concept of using a scale or weight as a measurement of success, because it's an arbitrary number. What does the number really matter if you're feeling great, you're happy, sleeping well, have great digestion, and your clothes are fitting you a little bit better. Isn't that a greater indicator of health and well-being than a number on a scale? Yes, I get it. Getting rid of the fat and losing weight is important, but not at the risk of your overall health and happiness, because let's face it, there is weight loss and there is fat loss. And, we know most people who focus on aggressive weight loss end up putting it back on because they haven't learned how to live a healthy lifestyle day by day.

Optimize!

For optimal health, it is essential that we pay attention and do the best we can in the areas of physical movement, sleep, nutrition, and stress management. Back in the day, when I was solely focusing on nutrition, I experienced limited success in truly helping people with their health and performance goals. The truth is, if I provided someone the best diet and exercise program in the world specifically designed for them, but if their sleep was compromised and they suffered from chronic low levels of daily stress, it simply did not work. Sure, they might lose some weight, but keeping it off is a different story. What is the point of losing weight if your health is compromised? Cardiovascular disease, autoimmune disorders and cancer do not care what you weigh.

When we have stress and we don't sleep well, our cortisol levels go up. Cortisol is the primary fight–flight stress hormone, which plays an essential role in our life. But, it can also be the root cause of many health issues, including undesired weight gain and undesired inflammatory conditions.

Understanding how industrialized, convenience-based, modern-day lifestyles affect our health, and we have to bring these things into balance. These are the primary pillars of health. You are what you eat; I'm sure you've heard that before. As humans, we are very physical creatures. Not even a hundred years ago, most people walked over five miles every day, for food, school, relationships, and work. Now, most people barely walk a quarter of a mile in a day. In addition to all of the walking, about 95 percent of the workforce was engaged in physical labor. Our sleep patterns were greatly impacted by the invention of electric lights and modern-day life is so stimulating that we can hardly calm our brains down, which causes stress, anxiety and lack of focus.

To best survive this environment, we need to adopt countermeasures to help create balance and calm down our nervous system. The goal is to create a balance between our innate humanity that has taken hundreds of thousands of years to evolve and the very new technologically advanced civilization in which we now find ourselves.

Don't get me wrong, we have accomplished amazing things over the past 100 years; but, it has happened so fast that we have not been able to keep up. Our bodies, brains and genes take tens of thousands of years to adapt to new stimuli. We evolved around nature, and now humans have created an artificial environment in which it's difficult to fully adapt. That being said, it's going to be a while before we can catch up to all of the technology, artificial light and chemicals that we have manufactured in recent years.

Acknowledging the fact that throughout all of human evolution we consumed natural nutrient dense foods, moved our bodies regularly throughout the day, went to bed with the moon and woke with the sun, and didn't have the constant mental stimulation that we are exposed to each moment of each day like we do now. To begin the process of creating balance, we first should identify the areas in our personal lives that are creating the most harm. I refer to it as addressing the "low-lying fruit," the easiest, most obvious things that we do, or shouldn't be doing, on a daily basis that are throwing us off kilter. We take an approach of slowly tackling one small, specific thing at a time, master it, and move on. Taking on too much, too quickly is usually a recipe for failure. I think most people reading this book relate to trying multiple times of doing too much, too quickly, and then finding out that it's not a sustainable process.

Real change takes time. True weight loss doesn't happen in a few weeks or months. Reversing disease is very possible, but it's not going to happen with pharmaceuticals. Real lifestyle change yields real health and performance results.

Now I will break down each of these four lifestyle components and provide a little more insight to why it's so important. Additionally, I will provide some quick tips and strategies to help correct your trajectory. Let's get started!

Nutrition

Definition: nu·tri·tion: the process of providing or obtaining the food necessary for health and growth.

Having good nutrition requires understanding the difference between feeding ourselves and nourishing ourselves. Our bodies are made up of approximately ten trillion cells. Each and every one of our cells is dependent on external factors. We have control over what we eat and drink and, to a certain extent, our environment (water, air, and dwelling). We make the choice every day to either consume nutrient-dense, real food, OR highly-processed, refined, empty calories.

We can have a direct impact on our cellular health. We can decide to either provide nourishment or withhold it. Disease is a form of cellular dis-regulation and dysfunction. This cellular malfunction is a result of what we're supplying and exposing them to. You are what you eat; we've all heard it, but it typically goes in one ear and out the other. We need to truly embody this concept, otherwise it's garbage in, garbage out. Granted, genetics also play a role, but the foods we eat have an epigenetic influence on them, which is the ability to influence or turn on or off certain genes and their influence on our physical body.

If we embrace this mindset and realize that certain things create more harm than good, we can really impact how we look, feel, and perform. Again, refined grains and sugars, as well as other types of manufactured, processed foods can be very addicting. Are we eating to self-medicate? In most cases, we are. We need to nourish ourselves rather than simply feed. Then, once we nourish ourselves, we start to feel much better. To be honest, most people don't know what it's like to feel good and have energy on a regular basis.

Poor energy levels often lead us to drink more coffee. And as good and potentially health coffee can be (in moderation) we are now overly dependent on it to mentally and physically function. Now because of this little habit, we're highly dependent and over-caffeinated. Then to make matters worse, we load it up with sugar, milk, cream or artificial creamers simply because most people can't tolerate the bitter taste of coffee. The result: We're drinking coffee for the stimulation but now we also have this sidecar of sugar and liquid calories on board.

This nutritional component is absolutely essential in order to maintain your health. There is no shortcut to good nutrition, but there are some strategies that can be very helpful. What we need to do is get back to some fundamentals so that we can more easily consume foods that are derived from real wholesome ingredients-- not processed, nutrient poor, refined foods that are loaded with preservatives and artificial colors and flavors.

All the food that we enjoy that comes out of a bag, box, or a drive-through window is laden with poor quality carbohydrates, proteins, and fat, slathered with flavor enhancers, salt and sugar in order to make it taste good. It's a societal issue. We fall into the mind set: "Hey, I'm on the road," or "I don't have time to eat." With that mindset, you end up consuming something that's quick and convenient albeit super tasty. Is it really, though? Once you develop the taste for real food, again, going back to the processed stuff you can actually taste the artificial and chemical aspects that are present. You'll also find that you're much more sensitive to the amount of sugar or salt that is in the manufactured, processed junk food.

Thirty plus years ago, with canned, frozen, convenient, and processed foods, we were sold a raw bill of goods: "Hey, why cook? Why go through all the trouble when you can eat this and go on about your day?"

Well, back then, that sounded great; freedom from the kitchen and no more having to clean up. We were even convinced that these manmade meals were healthier than the real foods that we had been consuming for hundreds of thousands of years. We were told that real fat -- saturated fat -- was the cause of heart disease and obesity. Real fat was replaced with highly refined manufactured fats, including so-called "vegetable" oils sourced from corn, soy, and canola. Those are all seeds by the way; they are not vegetables. So, do you think that we became healthier because of this shift? The answer is no, our health actually became much worse.

When this war on fat began, it was hypothesized that if we can cut out the real fat and replace it with vegetable oil (poor-quality industrial seed oils) then we would see a positive impact on heart disease, which was the number one killer at that point in time. These "vegetable" oils are now recognized as a cause of heart disease rather than being preventative. I mean, honestly, do you actually think that there is fat in corn? How in the world does one make oil from it then? Through a lot of heavy duty chemical and mechanical manipulation, that's how. Not with the intention of being repetitive, but I will be bringing this up again later in the book. I feel that it is that important for you to understand.

Additionally, the low-fat craze then led us toward eating more refined grains and sugars. Because of this we found that cardiovascular disease, diabetes, and obesity actually increased, not decreased, because of these nutritional practices. Certainly, we have raised the concern for cardiovascular disease; therefore, we are more diligent in looking for it as an early intervention. This is rarely treated with a nutritional intervention though; it is mostly addressed with pharmaceuticals even though the cause is mostly dietary. Yet, we still follow the same guidelines, low fat and the use of vegetable oils. We need to re-educate ourselves and society about nutrient-dense real foods that nourish rather than empty calories that can cause harm.

With convenience foods flooding our life, they have created an environment where we don't need to cook anymore. However, there are feasible strategies to employ, such as purchasing, prepping, and cooking in bulk. Getting used to the concept of leftovers is very helpful: prepping your vegetables and cooking in larger quantities, so that you have leftovers throughout the week. I know that it's not fun and exciting. It's certainly not as tantalizing as a trip to the drive-through. But again, if you want to nourish and thrive rather than simply feed and survive this is a powerful place to start.

Eat Your Vegetables!

If you're looking to nourish your body and rid yourself of excess pounds and disease, and perform at a mental and physical level that you've never experienced before, it starts with food. You have to fuel the body properly. In order to supply yourself with the right nutrients, You should start with consuming more vegetables. Let's consider the age-old question: "What's for dinner?" Typically it starts with a protein, right? We have chicken, beef, fish, pork et cetera. Add to that some form of carbs such as potatoes, rice or pasta. Vegetables are usually the last thing on our mind. It is often some form of guilt that leads to us putting it on our plate

My relationship with vegetables began with some form of overcooked canned vegetable that tasted terrible and was very mushy. Good quality, properly prepared vegetables, can be amazing! So, let's ask the question again: "What's for dinner?" Well, let's start with a vegetable. This could be a large salad or any other form of fresh or frozen vegetable. Focus on a wide variety and diversity. Broccoli can be very healthy, but if it's the only vegetable you eat day in, day out, you should attempt to diversify. The fact is that we don't eat nearly as many vegetables as we did in the past. Our ancestors ate far more vegetables on a daily basis, with a larger variety of colors and nutrient density.

Modern-day vegetables themselves can be an issue as well, especially if they're conventionally grown with the use of herbicides and pesticides. This is why organics are important to consider. Recent studies have shown that some of our modern-day health issues are a result of our exposure to the chemicals used in conventional farming practices. We need to focus on nutrient density and quality whenever possible. We do that by eating as many vegetables as possible, with a moderate amount of fats and proteins, and certainly keeping an eye on not only the quantity of our carbohydrates and starches, but the quality.

When it comes to nutrition, the typical "calorie-in-calorie-out" model has led to our unhealthy association with food. Calories do play a role, but there are more important aspects that should be made a priority. If a calorie's a calorie, then wouldn't it be fair to say that there is no difference between three hundred calories of butter vs. sugar vs. a piece of chicken? Those foods are very different from each other. It is my opinion that the quality of your food is more important to address first than the quantity.

If you address the quality of your food first you might be surprised at the results you might get. Then maybe address the quantity in order to fine tune your caloric needs. Unwanted weight gain, disease, and poor performance are greatly impacted by poor-quality foods. Processed refined foods cause hormone disruption, inflammation, and weaken the immune system. All which can lead to unwanted weight gain and illness.

Trust Your Gut

Another aspect that must be considered is that if you are what you eat, then your intestinal micro flora is also what you eat. Your gut biome, the three or so pounds of bacteria that live in your lower intestinal tract, is directly related to your mental and physical health. It has a significant influence on your immune system and mental health, as well as many other systems of the body. For those of you who are not that familiar with gut flora, you might have heard of probiotics or fermented foods, like yogurt that contain probiotics. These supplemental forms are intended to help support your already existing intestinal flora.

When we neglect to feed and nourish this organism properly, the downstream effect it has on us is quite profound. There are more than a thousand different species of bacteria that make up a population of around 100 trillion cells.

This super organism should act like an orchestra; be balanced and form a symbiotic relationship with your body and brain. When we don't feed ourselves right, our gut flora can become imbalanced causing what is referred to as dysbiosis – a leading cause of many common diseases and health issues, many of which are associated with your gut, but also several other physical and mental conditions not related to digestion. However, there are also several byproducts generated from your intestinal micro-flora. For instance, upwards of 90 percent of the serotonin in your body, a primary neuro chemical used in the brain that promotes a sense of wellbeing, is produced and stored by the bacteria in your intestinal tract. Another product called butyrate, which is very important for our health by providing much needed energy to the cells in the lower digestive system, aids against colon cancer, helps control inflammation and can positively influence the immune system.

In fact, research has suggested that upwards of 80percent of our immune system is regulated and modulated by our gut flora! We have to make sure we take care of this bio mass.

One of the big problems in modern society that can negatively impact this system is the overuse of antibiotics. Certainly antibiotics are meant to kill bacteria, but unfortunately it kills both the good and bad. Again, when we have a bacterial infection, antibiotics are typically used to kill the bad bacteria. Unfortunately, antibiotics also kill the good bacteria.

When we are born, our intestinal tract is a relatively sterile environment. Then, as we age, our gut is slowly populated with bacteria. The bacterial mass that develops helps shape who we are and helps establish the strength of our immune system. Our gut flora is as unique to us as our fingerprints. Our body develops a symbiotic relationship with it. Imagine that at three or four years old, you get an infection, and you take an antibiotic. Taking that antibiotic is almost similar to clear-cutting old growth forest. It cuts down all the beneficial bacteria and who knows what might grow back in its place. If you've ever seen a clear-cut forest, it doesn't grow back the way it was. It's overrun by shrubs and invasive plant species, which then create a completely different environment than what was there before. The same thing happens in our gut when we take antibiotics. Granted, antibiotics are imperative to our survival these days and have brought a significant increase to the quality of our lives.

In fact, there are certain situations where they can most certainly save your life, but the truth is that they are used much too often and for unnecessary reasons. In short, unnecessary over use of antibiotics has contributed to many modern-day health issues that plague our society

Your gut flora relies on what you feed it. This is another reason why we need to make vegetables part of our daily life. The fibers and starches that are in plants, from leafy greens to starchy roots and tubers, provide the optimal food for our gut flora. The fermentable fiber and resistant starches in real food do not get digested and enter the blood for our use. However, our gut flora utilizes them as the ideal food. These are referred to as "pre-biotics." It is important to make sure that we eat plants for not only their nutrient density, but also for the fiber and starches that allow our gut flora to thrive.

Carb Overload

Another very important situation that must be addressed is our dependence on highly refined grains and sugars--especially the impact that these foods have on our blood sugar. Before calories are even a consideration, we must acknowledge the hormonal impact that these products have on us. Believe it or not, our mental state can be easily "high-jacked" by rising and falling blood sugar levels. When our diet is high in refined carbohydrates (grains and sugars mostly), inflammation and hormonal chaos typically ensues. Many people subsist on these types of items consuming up to 60percent, 70percent or even 80percent of their calories from carbs alone.

There are people from different cultures around the world that can thrive on higher levels of carbohydrates. But, for most people, too much carbohydrate in the diet, especially the refined variety, poses a significant problem and health risk. Carbohydrates serve primarily as fuel for our cells. Think of it as gasoline for your car. A small to moderate amount is typically okay, but if we over-consume them on a regular basis, it can become problematic. Health issues such as diabetes, high cholesterol and triglycerides, unwanted body fat, fatty liver disease, and other metabolic and inflammatory issues are often as a result of the over consumption of carbs; especially refined carbs.

Many of us still carry the belief that eating fat can actually cause fat to accumulate in their body. Fortunately, it doesn't necessarily work that way. Yes, fat is high in calories and over consuming calories can be a problem. However, over-consuming carbohydrates can do the exact same thing and more. Our bodies need a certain amount as fuel, but if we "overfill the tank." our liver is then called into action in order to help sweep up the unused carbs in the blood stream. The liver then turns unused carbohydrates into triglycerides, cholesterol, and body fat.

This is a very simplified description of the process, but I think that it paints a clear picture of the fundamentals. In short, blood sugar regulation is a very important process and keeping this system functioning properly is essential for your health.

When we nourish ourselves with a balance of nutrient dense macronutrients (proteins, fats, and complex carbohydrates), we have a much better chance at regulating our blood sugar. When our blood glucose (sugar) levels are stabilized and we become more metabolically flexible (ability to efficiently burn fats, as well as glucose for energy) our bodies and brains function as they should. This way of eating also helps address metabolic disease and disorders such as type II diabetes and polycystic ovarian syndrome (PCOS). Fueling ourselves with the right macro and micro nutrients helps lower stress levels, improves mental clarity, provides more energy, reduces food cravings, and much more.

There is a long-running philosophy that states carbohydrates are absolutely essential in our diet. Although I am not what is referred to as a "low carber," we all must admit that most people over consume carbs, especially refined carbs, on a regular basis. The emergence of low carb/ high fat diets, have shown a lot of promise in treating several health issues. A diet structured this way is often referred to as a ketogenic diet and its premise is to have the body burn fat as its primary fuel source rather than carbohydrates. Although this can be an extremely effective practice, for most people it can be very difficult to sustain for the long term.

I typically utilize a low carb or keto diet for specific conditions or if the client has a particular goal. I do feel that there is a happy middle ground though. As I mentioned earlier, the body's ability to be metabolically flexible offers several health benefits. In fact, humans existed with this capability until it was lost through our over-consumption of industrialized of food, along with our addiction to sugar. The fact is that in today's environment most Americans are not adapted to burn fats as a fuel source very well.

Most people are primarily driven by carbohydrates as a fuel source. I think most people reading this have experience with cutting carbs and then feeling weak, getting headaches, and being irritable. In most cases these are the symptoms of a sugar crash and withdrawal. When we subsist on a high carb diet and then drastically reduce them, we can suffer from the dreaded "low carb flu." If you put a plan together that reduces the amount of carbohydrate and replace the "empty" calories with healthy fats, you'll find that you become more *fat-adapted*. That is, being able to burn fat more efficiently as a fuel source in addition to carbohydrates. This process initially takes about a week or two to occur--for some a little less and for others a bit longer.

Burning carbohydrates as a fuel is akin to burning paper. Alternatively, using fat as fuel is more like using coal. One burns very fast and hot, the other more slow and provides more sustained energy. In addition, there are significant cognitive benefits to burning fats as an energy source over carbohydrate. Personally, I'd rather be fueled by fats, because they last longer and don't bog down my brain like carbs and sugar do.

Micronutrients

Beyond our macronutrient (carbohydrates, proteins, and fats) intake, we need to assess the micronutrients that are available in our foods.

That's where smart supplementation can come in. I feel that nutritional supplements can play an important role regarding our health. About 10 years ago, or so, I believed that all of our nutrient needs could be met with an optimal nutrient dense real food diet; but for most, this is not feasible. Also, the nutrient density of many foods just isn't the same as it used to be. Soil health and the rampant use of herbicides and pesticides have created unfortunate results as it pertains to our food and environment.

For instance, let's consider the mineral magnesium. Magnesium is essential for hundreds of different types of metabolic and biological processes in the body, but over the decades it has been lacking in the standard American diet. One reason is from the lack of diversity in our diets; the other is because our soil has been depleted of this mineral from less-than-healthy agricultural practices. It has been clinically proven that magnesium supplementation can be very helpful and almost essential for many people. Not only is magnesium essential for energy production, but taking a 300 to 400 mg before bed can help you get better sleep and helps calm the nervous system.

Another example would be vitamin D3. Modern lifestyles have pushed us to spend more time indoors, especially in the winter. We also avoid the sun for fear of getting skin cancer. And if we do get outside, we typically slather ourselves with sun block to avoid the risk of getting burned or causing skin damage. These practices have led to a vitamin D3 deficiency in many people. In the winter months, especially if you live farther from the equator, supplementing with some D3 could be particularly helpful. Have your blood tested first before you start taking a D3 supplement, as your levels may be within the desired range. It is also important that if you do supplement your diet with D3, that you also consider taking vitamin K2. This is important because of their roll in calcium balance and utilization.

All that being said, magnesium and vitamin D3 deficiency are a big problem in modern society. For instance, let's look at osteoporosis. Most of us think of calcium when it comes to this condition, but believe it or not most of us have more than enough calcium in our diet and bloodstream to meet our needs. When D3 and magnesium are not in sufficient supply and/or out of balance, then our bone health can be compromised. D3 helps calcium get absorbed into the blood from the digestive system and magnesium is a key mineral when it comes to the formation of bone.

For a lot of people, taking D3 and magnesium could be just what the doctor ordered. In addition to bone health, both of these nutrients play a large role in several other areas of our overall health.

Fatty Acids

In addition to cleaning up our diet there are some nutritional practices and supplements available that are very beneficial to our health and help reduce inflammation. One that you might have heard of is omega-3 fatty acids. Omega-3s are polyunsaturated fats that primarily come from the ocean, sourced from cold water fatty fish and krill. There are also some plant sources, but the amount and form is not as rich as those that come from the sea. Omega-3s can also be taken in a supplement, in the form of pills or liquids.

I recommend omega-3s for my clients who suffer from chronic inflammation, are at cardiovascular risk, or are concerned with their mental health. They can also be taken if you are an athlete or are just interested in general health.

It is important to dose omega-3s appropriately based on your needs, so please consult a professional before adding this supplement to your daily regimen.

In addition to the negative impact that sugars and refined grains have on our health, there is something else that I feel could be even more detrimental to our health. One of the biggest issues with processed foods is the use of industrial seed oils, aka vegetable oils. As I mentioned earlier, corn is not as much a vegetable as it is a seed. The same goes for soy, canola, grapeseed, sunflower, and safflower.

These seed oils have infiltrated our food system and are a major cause of several health issues, mostly associated with inflammation. One particular reason is the fact that they are *processed* poly-unsaturated fats (PUFA's). This makes them more easily susceptible to damage from oxygen, light and temperature. All of which results in spoilage of the oils. Oxidized and potentially rancid fats are very unhealthy to consume.

An additional harmful aspect associated with these industrial oils is the amount omega-6 fatty acids that they contain. Omega-6's are not themselves harmful; in fact it's an essential nutrient that we require in our diet just like we require its more famous sibling omega-3. In fact, there are other omegas besides 3 and 6, such as 5, 7, and 9.

But unfortunately, because of the use of seed oils in food manufacturing, restaurants, and cooking oils, the intake ratios of these essential fats are greatly off balance. For example, if we went back a century or two ago, we would see that the intake of omega-6 to omega-3 fatty acids were on a ratio of about 3 to 1 respectively. But because of the high use of these seed oils in the food industry, our intake of omega-6 to omega-3 is more like a 20 to 1 ratio respectively. This nutritional imbalance is a powerful contributor to many diseases of oxidative stress and inflammation. One of the more common conditions is cardiovascular disease (CVD). It is important that you know that CVD is not necessarily a disease of high cholesterol, but a disease of inflammation! This is well supported in medical research.

Speaking of inflammation, this is a significant contributor to mental and physical illnesses. Granted, inflammation is actually necessary when it comes to physical injury or when an acute illness occurs. Unfortunately, many of us suffer from chronic low levels of inflammation because of less than ideal lifestyle choices. Poor-quality food, stress, and a lack of sleep all can contribute to low levels of unnecessary chronic inflammation.

Taking an omega-3 supplement or better yet, eating more cold water fatty fish improves that ratio by increasing our intake of omega-3. But, just as important (maybe even more so), is the lowering of the amount of omega-6 in our diets by eliminating these industrial seed oils from our home cooking, salad dressings, packaged foods, and restaurant meals. Greatly reducing our omega-6 intake can have as much of an impact as taking an omega-3 supplement.

If you are going to take an omega-3 supplement, I highly recommend you invest in a good-quality product. Do your research. You don't want to buy the cheapest one out there, because omega-3 fatty acids, being poly-unsaturated-fats, can oxidize and spoil very quickly. If they're not processed and packaged correctly, they can end up causing more harm than good.

I feel that some of the higher quality and more readily available omega-3 supplements on the market come from Scandinavia. You typically want to find one that is at least processed in an oxygen-free environment and is not heated. The brands available at your local pharmacy or box store typically do not use quality processing methods; which typically results in a poor-quality product that can actually be unhealthy. You might end up paying more for a high-quality product, but again, if you buy a substandard product, it can do more harm than good.

I highly recommend people do a little research and invest in a good quality omega-3 or fish oil if they feel that It would be helpful. However, it's also important to eliminate as much Omega-6 as you possibly can, that can also have a profound impact.

In short, getting rid of the foods that cause inflammation and eating more "anti-inflammatory" foods such as organic fruits, vegetables, herbs and spices. Focus on nutrient density and limit refined sugars and carbohydrates in your diet.

We get bombarded with information on what to do and what not to do on a daily basis. And, yes, all of this stuff can get very complicated, but it doesn't need to be. Keeping things simple and following the basic rules established by our ancestors is always a great place start. Practice the fundamentals in order to build a solid foundation and grow from there. Healthy practices can be a waste of time and money if they are applied to a weak foundation. This is why I not only practice nutrition, but also specialize in physical movement, sleep, and stress management. It's essential that we think of lifestyle practices as an orchestra: If one of the instruments is out of tune enough, it can throw the whole thing off.

Starting Tips:

<u>Don't Drink Your Calories</u>

If you feel that your nutrition situation is helpless, the best place is to start is to avoid any liquid calories such as juice, soda and sweetened tea. If you do consume juice and soda regularly, it is easy to slowly wean yourself off over a relatively short period of time. Sugar and caffeine addiction can be stressful to kick; but in about two weeks' time, it can be done. Substitute sugary drinks with seltzer or flavored sparkling water. If you must use an artificial sweetener, Stevia is probably the best choice. However, I also suggest that you try to avoid as many sources of artificial sweeteners as much as you can.

<u>Limit Packaged Foods</u>

Avoid most packaged foods as much as possible. Reduce or eliminate the sugar, refined grains, and industrial seed oils (vegetable oil) from your diet. You do not need to do it all at once: Simply start with a few key ingredients in your kitchen. Try to get in at least one nutritious meal each day. Avoid any unnecessary snacking and treats. Simply start with that. If you're still stumped, focus on dropping any soda, chips and sweets. Replace poor-quality seed oils with olive oil, avocado oil, good-quality butter (such as Kerry Gold) and coconut oil. There are healthier choices than seed oils available to you. Healthy fats that come from natural sources are very important, whereas most industrial seed oils can be extremely problematic

Better Breakfasts

I strongly recommend that people who suffer from metabolic disorders or blood sugar regulation issues assess their first meal of the day. If it is made up mostly of sugar and refined grains and lacks protein and healthy fats, this could be a significant area for improvement. Let me ask you this: How come it's easy for us to accept having breakfast for dinner, but the thought of having dinner for breakfast is frowned upon? Admit it; we have all had pancakes or waffles for dinner, right? But how often have you had chicken, salmon or steak with veggies or a large vegetable salad for breakfast? A typical American breakfast that leans more toward protein and fat would be bacon and eggs, right? Well, if you can't stomach the idea of having some chicken or fish for breakfast perhaps an omelet or frittata with a large portion of vegetables would be more acceptable.

Focus on more savory foods and more balance (protein, fats and carbs) in the composition of your breakfast. Again, most American breakfasts start off with something that is more like dessert than a nourishing meal. If you are tired of having low energy and constantly crave food or if you are a frequent grazer that feels the need to eat often, skip all that sugar and flour and try some real food

As an example, if you like hot cereal, omit the brown sugar and sugary fruits and try adding some seeds, nuts, unsweetened shredded coconut, ground flax seed and berries instead. I always have some organic frozen berries available that I can put into my hot cereal when I decide to have it. I try to make it more balanced; therefore, more complete. I'll even occasionally stir in some protein powder for good measure.

Snack Right

Remember to emphasize nutritionally balanced meals throughout the day, even when it comes to snacking. Some people consider an apple a decent snack. Yes, it can be; but by itself, it's all carbohydrate. It certainly contains nutrients and fiber, but lacks protein and fat, which are more satiating and help control blood sugar. Also, modern-day fruit is almost to akin to a candy in many cases. Most of the fruit available at your local market is grown to be larger and sweeter than what it used to be not too long ago. Before the emergence of commercial agriculture, fruit, in its natural state was smaller and very tart in taste. The carbohydrate or sugar in fruit is mostly fructose; therefore, too much fruit in one's diet can be problematic if you are looking to lose weight or if you have blood sugar issues. A smaller piece of fruit, balanced out with something like almonds or walnuts, can be a much healthier choice.

Hydrate

We all know that hydration is important for health, but how much water one needs on a daily basis to stay hydrated is very individualized. I recommend that you at least you start your day with a nice big glass of water and then drink more water when thirsty. Drinking too many fluids can actually over hydrate us. This can dilute the electrolytes in our system. A recent trend that has proven to be healthy is to add some fresh lemon juice to your morning glass of H2O. The notable health benefits are improved digestion, weight loss, improving the immune system and healthier liver function. Apple cider vinegar is another ingredient that could be beneficial. It can help you lower belly fat, control blood sugar, fight cancer and improve heart health. Both practices have been used for centuries in different cultures around the world.

For people who drink a lot of water, especially athletes or people working in hot environments, electrolytes are an important thing to be mindful of. When we sweat, we not only lose water, but also sodium and potassium, as well as other minerals. If we rehydrate with just plain water, we are at risk of diluting the electrolytes in our blood. This can negatively impact energy levels, induce muscle cramps and potentially affect your heart.

This is yet another reason for consuming plenty of quality vegetables and fruits in your diet. They contain the micronutrients that we need to function at our best by providing a wide variety of vitamins, but also the minerals potassium, magnesium, sodium, calcium, selenium, zinc, copper, iron, phosphorus and manganese.

The Timing of your Meals

One of the hottest nutritional practices out there right now pertaining to diet is the practice of intermittent fasting (IF) or time-restricted eating (TRE). Both of these practices are basically the same and address probably one of the most problematic dietary practices in our society: having too large of an eating window throughout the day. We spend more hours each day consuming food than we do sleeping, not allowing enough time for our body to recover, restore and repair itself. Spending more than 12 hours each day consuming food keeps our body from fully entering this restorative phase. Even with a disregard to the quality and the quantity of food, the window of time we spend eating each day dramatically impacts our health. If you consider the fact that there are 24 hours in a day, and if we are lucky enough to get the recommended eight hours of sleep each night, then potentially we could be spending up to 16 hours each day eating. Now I know that we take breaks between meals and snacks, but what we need to consider is the entire window of time each day that we are consuming food.

When we spend more than 12 hours each day consuming food, we're not giving our cells enough time to clean and repair and regenerate. When we're constantly bombarding our cells with food and calories, they are forced to constantly work and are not given enough time to recover. This is an important factor related to our health, body weight and disease.

By practicing IF/TRE, we allow our cells time to regenerate and clean up. The magic number is about 14 hours of fasting and a 10-hour window to eat. Typically, eight of those hours should be spent sleeping, leaving around six hours of your day "fasting." You can easily do this by stopping the consumption of food three to four hours before bed and waiting about two to three hours after you wake to begin again. I highly recommend that people stop eating around two to three hours before bed regardless, and not necessarily start gobbling down food as soon as they wake up.

Consider starting with a 12-hour fast, with a 12-hour window to eat. The real magic, though, happens at around a 14:10 ratio; 14-hour fast, and a 10-hour eating window. If you eat this way five out of seven days each week, you still reap the benefits but allow yourself a little more freedom on the weekends to enjoy spending time with friends and family without the worry of when you should or shouldn't eat. .

If you eat at the 16:8 ratio you can even expect better results. We're talking about further optimizing your health and well-being. IF has been proven to have a profound impact on longevity, fighting disease, cancer and inflammation. It helps to reset and balance our hormones, which then can have an effect on our metabolism and help with weight loss. The affect that I enjoy the most is the level of mental clarity and energy that I experience.

I think that, from a health and physical performance standpoint, IF/TRE is one of the most impactful dietary practices there is. And the best part, it's simple and doesn't cost a dime. In fact, it would probably end up saving you money. Believe it or not, our ancestors practiced IF/TRE all the time. Do you actually think that food was readily available every day of the year and that our ancestors ate in the dark? It is only in modern times that food has been readily available 24/7/365. And, I would like to argue that most of it isn't even real food!

To summarize: Focus on eating mostly when it is light out, and try and stop once it gets dark out. This practice can also have impact on your circadian rhythm and sleep quality. It's all in balance. If you eat closer to the cycles of the sun and avoid eating after the sun has gone down or before it's come up, it can positively impact your sleep patterns, as well. Now, doesn't that make sense?

Movement

Physical activity can be an effective tool for weight loss. I don't think anybody's going to argue with that. However, science has proven that about 80 percent of weight loss actually happens in the kitchen. In other words, it is your diet that will mostly dictate weather you lose or gain weight. Using exercise alone as a means for losing weight isn't necessarily the best approach. Unfortunately, exercise does not make up for an unhealthy diet. For example, doing an hour at the gym isn't going to negate the pizza, chips and soda you had for lunch no matter how many calories you burn. Yes, you can absolutely burn off the calories you consume, but exercise does not address the impact that poor quality foods have on your hormones, inflammation and immune system. However, the impact that physical activity and exercise has on your nervous system and brain is where the real magic happens.

I don't think that there is anybody in today's world who would say that they are absolutely stress free. If you have ever been a regular exerciser, I would bet that you would agree that being physically active on a regular basis makes you feel better, mentally and physically. Exercise as a means of dealing with stress is a very effective practice. In fact, humans have been practicing physical activity though out all of human existence.by walking, lifting heavy things and occasionally pushing the heart rate up once in a while. I'm not talking about in the gym. I'm talking about day to day life; walking up to 10 miles a day for work, food and family, building and manual labor and occasionally running for their life or chasing something down. Only in the past 100 years or so have we become so docile. And with lower levels of physical activity we have experienced a significant rise in mental health issues such as stress, anxiety and depression. A little bit of physical activity each day helps lower stress and increases one's ability to concentrate. It helps lock in learning, aids in digestion and promotes better sleep.

Also, exercise helps us maintain physical mobility. When I worked in the geriatric field early in my career, regular physical activity was essential to the daily lives of the residents. The number one cause of premature death, that's not associated with direct disease, is the loss of muscle mass and physical ability to get up and down from a chair, use stairs and walk moderate distances. Once one or more of these abilities are lost, then our quality of life and state of mind declines rapidly. Then, unfortunately, mental and physical disease sets in and in some cases we die younger than we need to.

Being physically active on a regular basis can help prevent mental and physical decline at any age. For children and young adults, it helps them maintain focus and aids in reducing negative behavior. If there are any video gamers reading this, you should know that regular vigorous exercise can help sharpen your reflexes and reduce fatigue. Just ask any pro video gamer about their physical fitness program and I am sure that you will be surprised to learn that they would say that they wouldn't be as good without it.

Obviously regular physical movement helps us keep our muscles, joints and ligaments tuned and more mobile. Humans are very physical beings by nature. As I mentioned earlier, if you go back in time to a hundred years ago, say before the invention of the automobile that, human beings walked a lot.; somewhere between five and ten miles each and every day. If you wear an activity tracker and are proud of the 10,000 steps that you get in each day, that's fantastic; but that's still only about half of the amount of walking that our great grandparents potentially did each day.

First and foremost, if you are not currently physically active, and even if you are, walking is just about the best activity that you can do. Humans are meant to walk, and not just to our refrigerators and back. Walking should be emphasized and practiced as much as eating food. It is that important. 30 minutes per day is a great place to start, and more is even better. If you have difficulty walking, it could very well be that it is a lack of walking that might be the cause. Isn't it funny how when people get older they stop doing certain everyday things such as walk or go up and down stairs? When it is quite possible that it is the lack of participating in those activities that could lead to that inability? Use it or lose it!

One of the main practices that has led to less walking has been the fact that we spend too much time sitting. Modern-day conveniences and the change in our work environment are to blame for this. For instance, those of you who might be reading this might be saying to yourself "My job requires me to sit at a desk," or "I spend so much time in my car, sitting at an airport or on an airplane." There are several things that can be done to counteract this. We need adopt daily countermeasures to combat all that chronic sitting. So, if you sit most of the day, are stressed out, carry too much abdominal fat or have a bad back, this is information is especially for you.

One thing that needs to be done is the opening of what are referred to as your hip flexors. These are muscles and tendons that make up the front of your pelvis. These muscles are part of the upper leg and lower abdomen. When we sit too much, this area gets very sort and tight causing a lack of mobility in your pelvic girdle; which, in turn, can cause a poor posture and back issues. When someone starts thinking about beginning an exercise program, running or jogging is quite common. There is nothing wrong with running, but if the body and mind are not prepared for it, it can become a great area of mental and physical stress. I believe that walking is enough for most people if done daily, but unfortunately society has pushed us to believe that we must push our heart and lungs to an uncomfortable level to achieve health. For optimal health, it is my belief, that everyone should walk at least 30-plus minutes every day as a foundation. From there, incorporate some resistance exercise 2 to 3 times per week and then work on getting in some cardiovascular work in 1 to 2 times per week. Anything more than that, I feel, is more performance goal oriented. A word of caution: please consult your doctor before starting any new exercises and if you plan on elevating your heart rate for any period of time.

Just as important, if not more, is the fact that we need to start moving more regularly throughout the day. This doesn't necessarily mean exercise, but just some physical movement sprinkled in throughout the day. This can greatly help negate the detrimental effects of chronic sitting. Another perspective that I would like you to consider is this, going to the gym regularly doesn't necessarily negate being inactive for most of the day. Yes, going to the gym can be great, but if you think that you are counteracting all of the sitting that you do, you're mistaken. We need to start breaking up the day into smaller segments and get in a little physical movement. Moving more throughout the day, in little bits and pieces, ideally every 30 minutes or so. Just stand and stretch for a minute or two. Take the stairs rather than the elevator, park farther from the door of whatever building that you might be going into. Something that is that basic and fundamental will make a significant difference over the years as we age.

The next step beyond basic regular movement and walking would be some form of resistance work. It is essential for us to do some form of strength exercise 2 to 3 times a week. It doesn't need to be that strenuous or complex. It can be simple bodyweight exercises, such as: push-ups, sit-ups, squats, pull-ups and lunges. You can use resistance bands, free weights or machines. It is imperative that we stress the skeletal–muscular system on occasion in order to maintain muscle mass and stimulate the nervous system. By activating the large and small muscle groups of the body we improve our physical and mental capabilities. My absolute favorite benefit that we get from vigorous exercise by far is the impact that is has on our nervous system. It can aid us greatly in our ability to mitigate stress and help us sleep better. It simply makes the brain feel good!

When it comes to cardiovascular work, everybody has their likes and dislikes, right? Running is a very simple exercise to go out and do. It certainly has its benefits, but if that's the only thing you do and you do it almost daily, it is very possible that you could be burning the candle at both ends. If you live with a lot of stress or have a mentally demanding job or lifestyle, high intensity cardio might not be the best choice. Doing chronic monotonous cardio exercises (such as using an elliptical, stationary bike, rowing machine or running) at levels that pushes your heart can have some benefit, but most of us over do it and actually are effectively throwing gas on our stress fire. Sure, it might feel good afterwards, but there very well could be some negative effects brewing as well. Ask yourself this, do you run or do any other form of cardio as a means of "self-medicating" in order to deal with your stress? If so, here is a word of caution. You could be putting yourself at a higher level of injury and/or cardiovascular risk. If you are a person that works and lives a very stressful life, try integrating in some strength work on occasion in addition to your cardio routine. Simply sub out a run or two each week and replace it with some strength exercises, you might be surprised at the results you get. And for any women that might be concerned that lifting weights will make them look bulky or put on too much muscle mass, don't worry. Gaining muscle mass is not an easy task to accomplish. It takes specific training and commitment to do so.

I'm more of a proponent, for general health, of doing cardio exercise about once or twice a week. Certainly, if you're a triathlete, runner or any other kind of endurance athlete, you're certainly going to need to do more than that. That being said, I <u>highly</u> recommend that all endurance athletes do some strength conditioning work as well. It will certainly improve your running, cycling and swimming abilities and help protect you from injury. As a cyclist myself, I only wish I found this out when I was younger: Doing things like dead lifts and squats have been fantastic for my own mental and physical performance ... an absolute game changer!

Again, the general formula is to walk every day, do some form of resistance work 2 to 3 times a week, and then elevate your heart rate maybe once or twice a week as a foundation. Again, please consult your doctor or health care professional before you engage in a new physical activity, to make sure that it's safe for you.

Starting Tips:

I think that wherever you are, if you're doing nothing right now, standing and walking more is a great place to start. Walking is and always will be the best activity anyone can do. It is unfortunate that most of us underestimate its effectiveness for health, longevity and wellbeing. If you are someone who is guilty of chronic sitting, this especially holds true. Too much sitting and inactivity is a major problem, not only physically, but also the impact that it has on the nervous system. Not enough physical activity causes a down regulation in metabolism.

So, to start, go for a 20-minute walk every day. That's it. Once you master 20 minutes, extend it to a 30 minutes. Walking daily and incorporating regular standing breaks could very well change your life. Use a timer to remind you to stand up every 30 minutes or so. If you spend much of your time at a desk on the phone, get a Bluetooth headset. That way you can walk around and spend more time on your feet. Standing breaks and regular movement every day throughout the day, over the years really adds up! People don't understand that health issues and disease are insidious. These little things, though you might not recognize the benefit today, tomorrow, next week or next month, will eventually have a huge impact over the years.

Once you master the walking and regular physical movement, try to start incorporating some strength activities. Such as pushups, body weight squats, sit-ups or other form resistance work exercises. Just mix it up and do a small variety of things that work different muscle groups. Personally, I am a big fan of yoga.

Then, if you can, get in some cardio work. Once or twice a week is plenty for most people. Shoot some hoops, kick a soccer ball around, play tennis or go for a jog. There are hundreds of options here. My only advice is to try and avoid doing just one thing, especially anything that is considered "chronic cardio." An example would be running on a treadmill for 30 minutes five days a week. It is certainly better than doing nothing, in most cases, but it can also be very limiting and potentially problematic.

As with all other areas of health and wellness, start out slow. Doing too much too quickly usually leads to failure. It is best to start with one simple goal, stick with it and master it. Otherwise, it puts too much stress on our already stressed body and mind. Real change takes time. Be patient with yourself, put in the time and work and then reap the amazing results. We are all aware of the practice of starting a New Year's resolution. The fact is that greater than eighty-five percent of all New Year's resolutions fail by the end of the first month. As an alternative, I implore people to adopt the practice of doing a "New Month's resolution."

Be it sleep, exercise, nutrition or mindfulness, practice one new thing each month and master it. Examples of this might be getting rid of liquid sugars/calories (soda, juice sweet teas) from your diet or going for a 20-minute walk each day. Master it, adopt it and bring it into your life making it a part of your lifestyle, just like brushing your teeth. Everybody brushes their teeth (or at least they should) everyday as a fundamental health practice. It's what we do. Well, we also need to be physically active every day in order to be healthy. There are no ways around it or shortcuts. It's just that we have made it too complicated and have developed a poor relationship with exercise, but it is fundamental to our human nature.

Most of this is so simple. You don't need a gym membership or fancy equipment. You only need some motivation to start. Walk and move daily, work your muscles 2 to 3 times per week and get your heart rate up once a week. The best way is to adopt more play and outdoor leisure activities in our life. That's it! Keep it simple and get it done. You will not regret it.

Sleep

Sleep, probably the most underrated and underutilized activity in our daily lives; a true superpower that can make or break us if not honored and used to its full potential. Unfortunately, most people neglect sleep and do not give it nearly as much credit as it deserves. How many of us have heard the saying, "I'll sleep when I'm dead?" Well, I promise you that with that mindset and practice you're probably going to end up dying much sooner than you might expect. Next to air and water, sleep is right up there as a necessity for life. We can only go a few minutes without air and only go a few days without water. But did you know that if you skimp on your sleep, your risk of death greatly increases, as well? As I have mentioned before, you could be practicing a healthy diet and exercise program, but if you're not getting adequate sleep, it's simply not going to work.

Studies have shown that if you get less than six hours of sleep, you are as impaired as someone who has had a few drinks of alcohol. A poor night's sleep can make you as insulin-resistant as a Type 2 diabetic. Sleep is the restorative process for the body and brain. When we sleep, everything changes in our system biologically. Sleep initiates metabolic waste clean-up, resets and balances our hormones, repairs damaged tissue including the rebuilding of muscle tissue from exercising. When we sleep; even the activity of our gut flora changes. Sleep helps reduces inflammation, strengthens the immune system and helps lock in learning. Your capacity to learn is only as good as the quality of your sleep. The better-quality sleep you get, the better you're able to retain information and learn. For athletes and gym goers who might be reading this, remember this, you are only as good as your ability to recover -- and that means sleep. As for intellectual and cognitive function, sleep is king for optimal performance. Sleep is absolutely essential for mental and physical performance. If you neglect or compromise your sleep, then you're constantly going to be struggling and find it difficult to achieve your goals.

The unfortunate reality though is that most of us neglect our sleep and subsist on sugar and caffeine in order to keep ourselves upright. Ask yourself this: What would happen if you couldn't have coffee for a week? If your immediate response is dread or panic, you might want to evaluate your sleep and dependence on caffeine. As a culture we subsist on Five-Hour Energy, Red Bull and coffee to keep the motor running. Thinking that it is creating more productivity and alertness, but none of those choices work nearly, as well as solid sleep. Now, some coffee or tea can certainly enhance your brain and energy levels, but is best when paired with quality sleep. Think of caffeine as an enhancement rather than a necessity. I promise you, that if you take a week or two, and you put some emphasis on your sleep before anything else, much of these other aspects of your life will become much easier.

As mentioned before, not getting enough sleep raises stress factors. Poor sleep causes a rise in cortisol levels, which is a primary stress hormone. Coffee on top of poor sleep can simply make matters worse. If you struggle to make healthy food choices or find it difficult get in daily physical activity because of low energy levels, I suggest that you start with evaluating your sleep.

For the majority of my clients, sleep is the weak link and is where I begin helping them regain their health and vitality. It really is the low-lying fruit that most people neglect. It has the greatest ROI amongst all other lifestyle practices. When we get good restorative sleep on a regular basis, the body and brain is ready to get up, move, make healthy choices and perform mentally and physically at a higher level.

Staying up too late with social media and movies while eating crappy food and possibly having a drink or two, greatly compromise our sleep. We then wake up in the morning, and start the process all over again. We eat something akin to dessert for breakfast, consume some form of sugary caffeine and hope that today will be better than yesterday. But, if we spend more time invested in getting better sleep, it can absolutely change your life for the better. Again, as I mentioned at the begging of this book, modern technology and advancements are amazing, but can also be a curse. As an example, let's consider Thomas Edison and his invention of the electric light bulb. As wonderful as electric light is, it can also cause significant health issues. Electric light allows us to stay up long after the sun has gone down, hence forever changing our patterns and disrupting our circadian rhythm.

For all of human existence up until about 100 years ago, all humans woke and slept in closer sync with the rise and fall of the sun. Now, with electric light, it is practically perpetual daylight. Electric light created the practice of shift work and working during the night. Unfortunately, this practice is one of the unhealthiest things we can do to ourselves from a health perspective. I highly recommend anyone who struggles with health issues and works the night shift strongly consider finding work that has normal daytime hours.

Studies have clearly indicated that shift work contributes to a much higher risk of developing disease and a shorter life span. It is imperative to not only get enough sleep, but to do so in sync with the rise and fall of the sun. Our relationship with the sun is as deep as our cells and genetics. All of life has a symbiotic relationship with the sun and to work against it will typically result in an imbalance in health. On a side note, we should all be getting daily sunlight exposure as well in order to help maintain a proper circadian rhythm as well as generate Vitamin D.

So, if a good night sleep aids in metabolic waste cleanup, cellular repair, hormone reset, lowers inflammation, protects mental health, memory and learning, doesn't it make sense to make it a priority in your life? As a health care practitioner, I emphasize sleep before diet and exercise; simply because a great diet and exercise program cannot make up for bad sleep, but great sleep makes eating a healthier diet and exercising much less toilsome.

Scientific evidence emphasizes that we should be getting between seven and nine hours of sleep each night. For those who get less than six hours of sleep each night or experience broken sleep, the first thing I would start with is making sure that what you do get is as solid as possible first and then try to elongate it.

There are some best practices to help you sleep deeper and longer. Start with making your room as dark as possible. Eliminate any sources of light and get rid of the TV in your bedroom. Watching TV in bed is a notoriously bad habit that impacts your health. If you cannot remove the electronics, try to cover them up. You can get an alarm clock that hides its display at night or use your smart phone as an alarm, just try not to keep it next to your bed. Any source of light can be very disruptive to sleep quality. Use blackout curtains, put some cardboard up or cover your windows with a blanket. Make sure that you are covering up all sources of light to the best of your ability and making your room as dark as possible. Try it for a week and see how your sleep can improve.

An even more impactful strategy to help improve sleep is consistency. Too many of us are going to bed at inconsistent bed times -- nine o'clock one night, eleven o'clock another. Just about every other aspect of our life is set to a schedule, why not our sleep? We are creatures of habit and we thrive on systems. We wake up at the same time. We go to work at the same time. We eat at approximately the same time. We do all these things systematically day in and day out, but when it comes to bedtime, we're all over the place. It is a much more natural practice to have a standardized bedtime. We do this with our kids, because we know the importance of sleep, but we then set horrible examples by staying up late and eating junk food. Once this irregular bed time sets in, we then cause a disruption of our circadian rhythm, which in turn is a cause of irregular sleep patterns.

It is also important to cut out as much of the blue light that we are exposed to the closer we get to bed time. Blue light from the morning and mid-day sun helps keep us alert and awake by influencing a rise in serotonin levels. Later in the day, as the sun goes down, the blue light that we are exposed to diminishes, lowering serotonin and causing a rise in melatonin. Throughout all of human evolution, the blue light that we have been exposed to has come from the sun. Today, however electronic screens emit the same blue light. Unfortunately, TVs, computers, smart phones and tablets are now one of the more prominent sources of blue light that we continue to use well after the sun has set. This negatively impacts our circadian rhythm, influencing serotonin to remain elevated and suppressing melatonin.

Reducing our exposure to blue light by limiting electronic screen use approximately two hours before bed would be ideal. If that is not an option and you <u>must</u> use electronics at night, consider looking into some form of blue-blocking technology. That could be an app on your computer, tablet or phone; however, you can also use a pair of blue light blocking glasses. I know plenty of people who use amber colored safety glasses that you can get from the hardware store for about $10.

Wearing them at night while using electronic screens helps cut the blue light frequency that enters the eye. It is the blue light entering the eye that influences our neurotransmitters related to our circadian rhythm.

Personally, I find reading as a great way to help fall asleep. Watching the 10 o'clock news just before bed, I feel is a less than ideal practice, because too much blue light emission and the downright depressing subject matter in most cases. This is not necessarily the best way to end your day.

Recap

The top tips for optimal sleep are:

- Blacking out your bedroom

- Maintaining a consistent bedtime

- Limiting the amount of blue light exposure two hours before bed

- Avoid eating or consuming alcohol two hours before bed

We need to pay more attention to when we are going to bed and the environment where we sleep. It is such an essential part of our rest, recovery and restorative process.

Our effectiveness during the hours that we spend awake are purely dependent upon our sleep quality and quantity. If you're dealing with weight issues, and you think you have a good exercise and diet program, but you can't seem to lose those last 10 pounds, I can almost guarantee that it's associated with poor quality sleep and quite possibly the amount of stress in your life.

Stress Management

Stress is something that we all experience almost on a daily basis. For some this stress is worse than for others. Truthfully speaking, stress is actually a good thing. It helps us develop mental and physical resilience. For instance, physical stress (jogging and lifting weights) help make us physically stronger. Whereas certain forms of mental stress help make us more mentally resilient, the truth is, these stressors should be intermittent and temporary. Unfortunately, in our current modern-day environment, stress is constant and unrelenting. Stress that makes us stronger typically comes from external influences, but most of today's stress comes more from our internal environment. In other words, the bulk of the stress that we face today is a result of our own thoughts.

The stress of days past was meant to spike and then quickly diminish. The stress that our ancestors faced was that of basic survival. It was not caused by financial or social concerns. Back in the day, if a bear was chasing us, we would run and climb up a tree in order to get away. This would cause a temporary spike in the stress hormone cortisol and then after some time, once the threat was gone, cortisol would then diminish. That is not the case today. Today, cortisol shoots up and stays up much longer than it should. Granted, if I am in a car crash I want cortisol to spike, it could very well save my life. But if my cortisol is spiking because my boss just yelled at me or if someone said something on social media that I didn't like or my bank account isn't as high as I would like it, that's not good at all and serves no purpose pertaining to health and happiness.

In this modern-day world, we are so hyper-stimulated and bombarded many different complexities of life. This causes our stress and our cortisol levels are constantly spiking without completely subsiding. Unfortunately, this situation often results in the use of drugs, alcohol, cigarettes and junk food in order to help us relax. The use of these substances cause a dopamine response in our brain and pushes cortisol to the side, temporarily. Dopamine is the primary "feel good" hormone in the brain and helps you feel relaxed and happy. We are so dopamine deprived due to lack of natural sources of stimulation these days that our desire for it is one of the leading causes of addiction.

We constantly worry about finances, relationships, work, and our children. We're constantly being bombarded by social media, advertisements and thoughts of food. It never stops. It's relentless. Then we're sitting there, wondering why we're overweight, sick, out of shape and unhappy.

Believe it or not, our mental health and ability to ward off stress begins with the three topics that I have already discussed: nutrition, physical movement and sleep. When any or all of those areas are compromised, we can easily suffer the mental consequences. For example, the mental strain that blood sugar swings create, or the impact that exercise has on the nervous system and certainly the negative impact that a single night, never mind years, of poor sleep can have on our health. Approximately 90 percent of all negativity that we face on a daily basis comes from our own thoughts. We need to practice strategies that help slow down our racing mind. We should try to incorporate a small bit of presence/mindfulness into each day to help combat the relentless stressors and senseless over-stimulation of everyday life.

When it comes to the act of practicing, mindfulness can take many different forms. Regardless of how you practice mindfulness, there are some of you that will find it almost impossible to accomplish, at first anyway. For many of us the mind is constantly processing and thinking to the point that we are never really aware of the present moment. One question that you can ask yourself is: "Do I feel comfortable being by myself in a totally quiet place?" I have found that for those who might answer that question with an absolute "no!" that they are the ones who might benefit most from a mindfulness practice. But really, daily mindfulness and meditation is for everyone. Those who practices mindfulness on a regular basis often experience fantastic results that can lead to lower levels of stress, a drop in blood pressure and a reduction in pain and discomfort. Another benefit is improved attention, concentration and memory.

In my work with corporate professionals, when I propose the concept of "surrender" or slowing down, relaxing or taking it easy, it is obvious that it is not typically in their nature. When we do decide to relax a bit, sometimes we can feel that we're going to be missing out on something or miss an opportunity, or that someone else is going to get ahead of us. The bottom line is that life is very long and wonderful, but unfortunately, we spend too much time worrying about little things that do not really matter. If we acknowledge at the generalities around stress and depression, we discover that stress is usually associated with worrying about the future, and depression is usually associated with thoughts and regrets of the past. Now granted, there are legitimate cases clinical depression as a result of biological imbalances or from traumatic experiences, but most cases of depression are not as severe and can be greatly improved with the right lifestyle changes. Clinical research has clearly identified systemic inflammation as a primary cause of most cases of depression and anxiety.

When we are trapped in thought and not paying attention to the present moment, many of these thoughts, especially negative thoughts, have a downstream effect to the rest of the body. Here is an example of why many people stress eat: Stress raises cortisol levels, our primary fight-or-flight hormone, and nearly all hormonal reactions create a cascade influencing other hormones. When one hormone goes up or down, it affects other hormones. If we have high stress, high cortisol, this causes glucose rise, but also reduces the amount of insulin released. Insulin is essential for glucose (blood sugar) metabolism. By understanding this it is easier to see how stress can lead to undesired weight gain. But it also can cause high blood pressure and be a key factor in other diseases. Also, when we experience this rollercoaster of hormones, we tend to want to eat, and in this case, highly refined carbohydrate and sugary products. Then we wonder why we can't make healthy choices. Stress and sleep are huge regulators for our hormones, which can then cause us to make poor dietary habits. Stress is a significant cause of disease and poor health.

I personally experienced this back in 2007-2008. My perceived life at the time was causing me high levels of stress and depression that eventually led to me getting sick and injured. Fortunately, I was able to turn my life around and began to make some simple lifestyle changes. I was surprised at how quickly my mental and physical health returned once I began to take care of myself, but I could easily see myself slipping back into some old habits. This is where my meditation practice came in. It helped me "rewire" my thought process and allowed me to become more responsive rather than reactive to the external world. This is coming from someone who's been an on-and-off meditator since the early nineties. I had to step back and reinvent myself. Questioning my objectives, goals and life's purpose as it pertains to me and my family's happiness and health.

Realizing that the mindfulness component was the greatest tool I have readily available to me, this is where I started manifesting the real change that I needed to be the best father, husband and overall human being I could be. I feel that a regular mindfulness practice has the greatest ability to help us make better choices and see the world from a better frame of mind. We need to discover and practice the methods that allow us to slow down the monkey mind, the mental movies and the "what-if" scenarios that plague us constantly. We're perpetually caught in daydreams.

Granted, we need to think in order to solve problems, be creative and engage with others, but most of my problems have always been solved when I take the time to quiet my mind. This is when most solutions arise to the tough questions that we face. When there are no other thoughts or external stimulus bombarding us. How do you solve a problem when you're constantly thinking about a problem? Sometimes you need to step away from it for a bit in order for the answer to arise. We only do that when we're living in the moment, fostering mental clarity.

You'd be surprised how something as simple as your breath can be used as a tool to improve your sense of mental and physical wellbeing. It can also teach you how to appreciate the moment and capitalize on the opportunities that are here and now. Most of us are too wrapped up in our thoughts to see what's going on in the present moment.

I frequently engage with individuals who think that meditation is not for them or that it has some type of religious connotation. I've come across my share of corporate professionals who, as soon as I mention the word meditation, they roll their eyes, and they're like, "Oh boy, here we go." But once I share with them the number of professional athletes', corporate professionals and Fortune 500 CEO's that have a daily mindfulness practices, they start to pay a bit more attention.

There are so many resources available to you and a multitude of methods to try. There's no one right way to do it. You could be playing tennis or knitting or lying down on the grass. Heck, I do it while I'm driving my car. Focusing on the in and out flow of my breath. It can be quite soothing.

On that note, breathing is one other significant resource that we can tap into in order to improve our mental and physical health. Believe it or not, most people have lost the ability to breathe properly. This is mostly due to chronic stress and too much time spent sitting. Both of these cause us to adopt bad breathing mechanics or poor breathing techniques that lessen the activity of the diaphragm muscle and lower lobes of the lungs. Using breathing exercises as a form of mindfulness and stress-reducing techniques is extremely effective. I personally do them almost every day.

If you're not necessarily in tune with the idea of meditating, then I highly recommend you research and do what's referred to as "diaphragm breathing exercises." Learning how to better activate the diaphragm and practice deeper abdominal belly breathing rather than short upper chest breathing or "sipping." For me, abdominal breathing exercises helped me lower my stress levels and enabled me to better relax my body and mind. It works like magic in helping me get back to sleep after waking in the middle of the night as well.

Reactivating a sluggish underused diaphragm is essential for our mental and physical health. Yes, we must use it in order to breath, but we don't necessarily use it as well as we should. We simply don't use it to its full capacity that is for sure. You'll be surprised on how effective proper breathing mechanics can help lower stress and anxiety. Breathing correctly and utilizing certain breathing techniques can help take you from being in a stressed-out fight-or–flight condition to more of a rest-digest and chilled out state of mind. We know that stressful events causes our nervous system to have a sympathetic response, but when we practice some very simple breathing techniques, we encourage the body and brain to switch to a more parasympathetic condition; which in turn reduces cortisol levels, anxiety and inflammation. This also fosters a more relaxed state of mind and happiness.

Starting Tips:

Probably the most important ritual that I try to do each morning is about ten minutes of yoga followed up by twenty or so minutes of meditation. Thirty minutes is a small commitment, especially when the return on the investment can save you hours of frustration and discontent throughout the rest of the day. You certainly do not need to start with that much time: five minutes alone of a simple mindfulness practice can have remarkable results. I suggest doing this first thing in the morning before you start your day. This is because as fantastic as practicing mindfulness in the evening can be, in some cases it is used to destress. But a morning practice can help ward of daily stress before it even begins. It's kind of like taking an aspirin for a headache. Wouldn't it have been better to prevent the headache to begin with? If we practice mindfulness in the morning, we have a greater sense of well-being as we walk into our day. We foster a better sense of mental well-being. Therefore, we're doing preventive maintenance rather than using meditation as a form of treatment. Granted, I am also a fan of evening meditation, but if I were only able to choose one I would do it in the morning. Simply start with a couple minutes each morning if possible, doing either some form of diaphragm breathing exercise or a more traditional mindfulness meditation practice.

There are some very effective resources available to you in from books, podcast and meditation apps on your phone. Speaking of apps, a few great ones to start with are *Headspace* or *Calm*. Both are fantastic for teaching people the fundamentals of meditation. Another one that I like very much is called *Oak*. This one not only provides effective guided meditations, but also has a set of great breathing tools.

If you deal with a lot of stress and/or anxiety issues, I highly recommend that you do NOT start your day looking at your phone. Jumping into email, news or social media first thing in the morning is a surefire way of turning on your sympathetic nervous system and starting your day with a mind full of worries, negative thoughts and distractions. You're being thrown right into the chaos, and once that has occurred, it is very difficult to turn off. You have a very important choice to make each morning. You can either start your day with a smile and a sense of ease or with mental distractions, anxiety and stress.

Another effective practice to do in the morning is keeping a journal, sometimes referred to as a gratitude journal. Either way, the act of writing down your thoughts and worries is an effective method of helping you work out your problems and declutter the mind. By listing a few simple things that bring you joy each morning has been shown to help foster more happiness and reduce stress. Just wake up in the morning, make your morning beverage, sit down, do some breathing exercises for a few minutes and then take out a piece of paper or journal and write down three things you're grateful for. They don't need to be complex. It could simply be that it's sunny out, or a beautiful sounding bird that you hear outside of your window. It could even be that delicious cup of coffee that you are sipping on. The fact is it doesn't really matter what it is as long as it makes you happy and are grateful for it. When you are thinking and writing about something positive, try to embody it. Carry the emotional response into your heart, feel it. Whenever I do this I can actually feel my blood pressure lower and my muscle relax. Simply feeling your observations of something as simple as the smell of fresh air or the feeling of the warm sunlight on your skin is so therapeutic. When we flood our body with nurturing thoughts, they then lead to a release of positive hormones and neurotransmitters that make us feel good and are extremely healthy for us. Alternatively, the opposite happens when we have negative thoughts and emotions, they end up causing discomfort, unhappiness, stress and potentially disease.

A couple of great books that I recommend are Eckhart Tolle's *The Power of Now* or Jon Kabat-Zinn's *Wherever You Go, There You Are*. These books can help you nurture and foster sense of well-being and peace in your world, rather than the competitive nature and sense of discontent that most of us live with on a day-to-day basis. Happiness is a choice. You simply need to begin to foster it a little bit each day. It will take time and patience, but the reward is very much worth it.

How to Get the Most Out of Your Body and Mind

When I start working with someone, it always starts with a series of conversations. When working with me, or any other healthcare professional, it is essential that you get to know each other beyond statistics and surface observations. It doesn't take very long to discover what each person is about and to start developing a good relationship that you feel comfortable with. Taking one step at a time and slowly developing new ways to look at and deal with the challenges of everyday life.

It is really a personal preference, but in my experience, if you want to create real long lasting change, the best way is to take it slow and master one small step at a time.

I like the concept of adopting a "new month's" resolution rather than a "New Year's" resolution. That way by the end of one year, you could potentially have 12 new lifestyle practices that you have mastered. That is much better than one massive lofty goal that will more than likely flop by the end of the first few weeks.

When working with individuals I utilize all of the data available to me, such as lab work, blood chemistry and genetic testing. I obtain a health history form, wellness logs, food intake, sleep data and assess your physical activity. I like to get a sense of what your day-to-day life is like and start identifying the "low-lying fruit." Sometimes the simplest little changes can yield some significant fast results. That is, any obvious thing that you might be doing on a regular basis that might be keeping you from achieving your goals. I typically don't use a big hammer to sledge out big results; those methods never last very long and usually cause unintended stress. I employ a much more systematic approach. It is best to choose one or two smaller things at a time that can yield positive results without evoking stress.

Starting slowly isn't always easy, but it doesn't take much time before momentum is created and things start to pick up. Once you realize how easy it is to make a change, faith and confidence grows and our ability to tackle bigger challenges improves.

Alternatively, when we attempt to take on too much too quickly, stress and anxiety set in; and before we know it, we find ourselves back where we began.

To get started, you have to understand that change takes time and patience and that there is no magic bullet to real long-lasting health and wellbeing. You have to be compassionate with yourself. You have to break down your concerns and goals into smaller more manageable pieces. This allows you to facilitate the change slowly and identify the true areas of concern. If you are saying to yourself that you would like to lose some weight, but the real problem is that you're not sleeping very well, a change in your diet and starting an exercise routine might not be as effective as you had hoped. Sure, you might drop a few pounds initially, but it doesn't take long for a plateau to occur and the frustration to begin. You need to fix your sleep first, then you can see how much easier it can be to eat correctly and be more physically active. We need to identify those primary areas because sometimes our goals are high jacked by hidden factors that we're not aware of or paying attention to.

By looking at our nutrition, physical movement, sleep, and stress management strategies individually we have a better chance a creating real change. It is often that one of those areas can easily take a back burner while the more pressing matters are addressed. Typically one area stands out more than the others and addressing it in small steps might not be glamorous or what everybody else is doing, but this is how real change occurs.

When it comes to nutrition, start with cutting down on refined grains, sugar and industrial seed oils. Artificial ingredients are never any good for us either. Start making a habit of reading ingredient labels. Feeling overwhelmed already? Then let's simplify it even more. How about just cutting the sugar out of your coffee or reducing the amount of soda you drink each day. One can of soda each day can equal up to five pounds of body fat over the course of one year, not to mention the impact that it can have on blood sugar swings and the inflammation that it can cause. That alone is a great place to start.

Once we start to identify some of the concerns under each topic, you should write them down. Don't try to stuff everything in your head and remember it all. Get a notebook and write things down, worries, needs, goals and observations. As I mentioned earlier, keeping a journal or log is a powerful tool in helping you address and meet your goals. Take it one day at a time, or maybe one month at a time. Try using the *new month's resolution* perspective towards your objectives. Remember, if you try to take on too much too quickly, then you can very well create more problems than solutions. Pick that one thing and be diligent about it, create a level of change that doesn't disruptive your life.

Once you realize that the changes you've made are effective enough to address your goals, yet subtle enough as not to disrupt your social life, then they seem much more doable and easy to maintain. In fact, over time, you might actually see that your friends may start making healthier choices as well. Once they see how easy it can be.

It is well known that change is hard and can be challenging for people. There's often no immediate reward associated with it. We are so accustomed to immediate results. Like taking a medication for a condition, the results can be amazingly quick. Like when you have a headache and how quickly it will go away when you take some ibuprofen. Or when we're stressed out and how impactful a drink or a pint of ice cream has on our sense of relaxation. Sure, in that moment, we are satisfied; but the effect is fleeting and never lasts. We always find our problems returning and having to deal with them over and over again. We have temporary solutions to conditions, but they never do last for very long. This is because we are only treating the symptoms and not the causes.

Real lasting, lifelong change is not always easy to accomplish. This is because, at times, it can be difficult to notice the results of our hard work; leading to frustration and eventually quitting. But with patience, time and compassion for yourself, these changes can have a significant impact on not only your life but also the lives of the people around us.

I find most people will be bystanders when it comes to their health. They know what they need to do, but they don't take action. I'm asking you to take action, but not to the point where you feel overwhelmed and frustrated. Find one small thing and start making a change today and build from there.

If you'd like my help, send me an email at **mattkansyrd@gmail.com**. I'd love to hear how this book has impacted you and what changes you've made in your life as a result.

Thank you!

Notes, Thoughts & Ideas:

Here's How to Get the Most Out of Your Body and Mind

Are you frustrated with how you look, feel and perform? Are you tired of not having enough energy? Unfortunately, there are no magic bullets out there when it comes to health and well-being, but real solutions are right at your fingertips. Unfortunately, most modern-day health issues are dealt with by treating the symptoms, not the root cause. And the root causes are often associated with our lifestyle choices. What we eat, our physical activity, how we sleep, and the stress that we experience.

That's where I come in. I help people just like you figure out what aspects of your life have the greatest impact on your health, happiness and performance, as well as, where to start and how to track the changes that will yield the greatest results in the shortest period of time.

Step 1: Identify your biggest challenges, align them with your goals, simplify the process and tackle one step at a time. This is how real lasting change occurs. As long as you're pointing in the right direction and consistent, in time, you can have fantastic results that will carry with you for the rest of your life.

Step 2: Start to act by addressing the single most obvious issue. Simplify it into smaller steps and take action. Don't try and do too much too soon or it could result in you falling back to your old habits. Most practices fail because of trying to do too much at once.

Step 3: Have patience. Your issues and concerns didn't occur overnight therefore you won't resolve them overnight either. Consistency is the key to long-term success. Don't beat yourself up if you miss a work out or eat something you shouldn't have. Acknowledge the slip, learn from the experience and get back on track.

Most people know what they need to do to be happier and healthier, but very few actually take action. Now with the right guidance and coaching you can create a new trajectory towards a healthier and happier life.

If you'd like my help, send me an email at: **mattkansyrd@gmail.com** and I'll take it from there.